HOW TO START WEIGHT LOSS ROUTINE

THE ULTIMATE GUIDE TO A HEALTHY BODY

Jeanelle K. Douglas

Contents

Table of Contents

INTRODUCTION

A woman named Jane lived in a bustling metropolis filled with the smells of freshly made coffee and the sounds of traffic. Jane was a lively person who was always up for a new adventure. However, in the rush and bustle of her everyday life, she began to struggle with her weight.

Jane recognized she wasn't comfortable in her own flesh when she looked in the mirror one morning. Her energy was low, and her confidence was waning. Determined to make a difference, Jane embarked on a weight-loss adventure. But where to begin? The vast amount of information accessible online and in periodicals overwhelmed Jane. Fad diets offered quick answers, while popular training regimens promised spectacular results. Jane felt lost and dejected, unsure of which course to choose.

While visiting a bookshop, Jane quickly picked up the book titled **"How to Start a Weight Loss Routine"** and began reading it. She took it and started reading because she was intrigued. The book attracted her with its complete weight reduction guide, realistic nutrition and exercise advice, and long-term maintenance tactics.

As Jane read more, she found herself nodding in agreement with the book's thoughts and counsel. She learned the value of setting realistic objectives, creating a supportive atmosphere, and the impact of mentality on attaining success. Jane felt more powerful and driven to take control of her health as she flipped the pages.

Jane ended the book with the information and skills she needed to begin her weight-loss quest. Jane went out to put the book's suggestions into action, armed with a renewed sense of purpose and resolve.

Months passed, and Jane's efforts were successful. She lost weight, acquired strength and confidence, and, most significantly, changed her lifestyle for the better. Jane's path was not without hurdles, but with the help of the book, she overcame them with tenacity and perseverance.

When Jane reflected on her journey, she recognized how much **"How to Start a Weight Loss Routine"** had influenced her. It was more than simply a book; it was a guide to a better, happier version of herself.

If you're at a crossroads in your weight reduction journey and don't know where to start, let **"How to Start a Weight Loss Routine"** guide you. This book is more than just another weight reduction guide; it is a buddy who will be by your side every step of the journey. From understanding the science underlying weight reduction to practical advice on nutrition, exercise, and lifestyle changes, this book provides a detailed road map to success.

This book is for you, whether you're a beginner ready to start your weight reduction journey or a seasoned veteran searching for new ideas and motivation. Allow it to be the spark for your transformation, directing you toward a better, happier, and more satisfying existence. With perseverance and devotion, you, too, can begin on a path of self-discovery and development. The trip starts right now.

Go get your Note Pad

Lets get to work

Chapter 1: Understanding Weight Loss.

Understanding weight loss

Weight loss is a multifaceted process that entails more than just losing extra weight; it is a comprehensive strategy for enhancing overall health and well-being. To begin on a successful weight reduction journey, you must first grasp the underlying systems and variables that influence weight development and loss.

The balance between energy intake and expenditure essentially determines weight reduction. When the amount of calories ingested exceeds the number of calories burned via physical activity and metabolic processes, the body converts the surplus energy to fat, resulting in weight gain. When energy expenditure exceeds energy intake, the body uses its fat reserves as fuel, causing weight loss.

However, the calculation is more complex than just comparing calories in and calories out.

Many additional factors influence an individual's ability to lose weight efficiently. Genetics, metabolic rate, hormone levels, sleep quality, stress, and underlying medical issues are all aspects to consider.

Genetics can incline people toward specific body types and metabolic patterns, impacting their ability to acquire and lose weight. The pace at which the body burns calories at rest, known as metabolic rate, varies across individuals and can have an influence on weight loss attempts. Insulin, leptin, and ghrelin are essential hormones that regulate hunger, metabolism, and fat storage, all of which have an impact on weight control.

Diet, exercise, sleep, and stress management are all important lifestyle variables that impact weight reduction. A well-balanced, nutrient-dense diet supplies the body with critical nutrients while promoting appropriate metabolism and energy levels. Regular physical exercise not only burns calories, but it also boosts metabolic health, muscular tone, and general well-being.

Quality sleep is critical for controlling hunger hormones, lowering cravings, and promoting a healthy metabolism and weight management. Chronic stress can cause emotional eating, disturb hormone balance, and promote fat accumulation, thwarting weight reduction efforts.

In addition to comprehending the physiological components of weight reduction, it is critical to grasp the psychological and emotional variables that might influence one's ability to begin and maintain a weight loss regimen.

Many people suffer from emotional eating, which is when they use food to cope with stress, boredom, melancholy, or other negative feelings. Addressing these emotional triggers and devising alternate coping techniques is critical for breaking bad eating patterns and creating a positive connection with food.

Mentality is critical to the success of a weight-reduction journey. A good attitude, establishing reasonable objectives, and staying motivated are essential components of a successful weight reduction program. It is critical to approach weight reduction with patience, tenacity, and openness to learning and adapting along the way.

Social and environmental variables might have an impact on eating choices and physical activity levels.

Surrounding oneself with a supportive network of friends, family, or peers who promote healthy behavior may significantly boost motivation and accountability.

Creating an atmosphere that promotes healthy living, such as filling the kitchen with nutritious meals, arranging regular exercise sessions, and limiting exposure to bad temptations, can all help with weight reduction.

Understanding weight reduction requires taking a holistic approach that tackles both the physical and psychological components of the process. Individuals may lay the groundwork for a successful and long-term weight reduction regimen by learning about the elements that drive weight loss and taking a holistic approach to health and wellness.

The Science of Weight Loss

The science of weight loss is founded on the fundamental principles of human biology and metabolism. At its foundation, weight loss happens when the body expends more energy than it eats, resulting in a calorie deficit and a fall in body weight. This approach is generally known as the "calories in, calories out" principle.

To further comprehend this theory, consider that the body requires a specific amount of energy to perform basic physiological activities such as breathing, digesting, and circulation. The basal metabolic rate (BMR) refers to the basic level of energy consumption. Physical activity and exercise also contribute to energy expenditure, as does food's thermic impact, which is the energy necessary for nutritional digestion, absorption, and metabolism.

When people consume more calories than their body needs for these tasks and activities, their bodies deposit the surplus energy as fat. When people consume fewer calories than their bodies require, the body begins to burn stored fat for energy, resulting in weight loss.

However, weight reduction results are influenced by more than just the number of calories ingested and spent. The quality of calories, or the macronutrient content of the diet, also has a substantial impact on weight reduction results.

Studies have demonstrated that protein-rich meals increase satiety, lower hunger, and boost thermogenesis, all of which aid in weight reduction and lean muscle mass retention. Similarly, fiber-rich diets based on fruits, vegetables, and whole grains might increase feelings of fullness and control blood sugar levels, perhaps aiding in weight management.

Furthermore, hormonal modulation of hunger and metabolism is crucial for weight reduction. Hormones, including insulin, leptin, ghrelin, and cortisol, work with the brain to control appetite, satiety, and energy expenditure. Variables such as nutrition, stress, and sleep patterns frequently impact these hormones, leading to disruptions in weight control and difficulties in weight management.

Understanding the science of weight reduction necessitates grasping the complex interaction of energy balance, macronutrient composition, and hormone regulation. Individuals may use this information to establish a weight reduction routine, allowing them to make informed food and lifestyle choices that support their objectives and encourage long-term success.

Furthermore, meal time and frequency might affect metabolic rate and weight reduction results. According to some research, intermittent fasting, which involves cycling between eating and fasting times, can help with weight reduction and metabolic health by boosting fat burning, insulin sensitivity, and growth hormone levels.

Furthermore, the makeup of the gut microbiota, a colony of bacteria that live in the digestive system, has emerged as an important factor in weight control and metabolic health. An imbalance in the makeup of the gut microbiota, known as dysbiosis, has been linked to obesity and metabolic diseases. As a result, techniques for fostering a healthy gut microbiota, such as eating prebiotic-rich foods and taking probiotics, may help with weight reduction.

Furthermore, it is critical to understand the idea of individual heterogeneity in weight reduction. Genetics, age, gender, metabolic rate, and underlying health issues can all impact how people respond to food and lifestyle changes.

For example, some people may have a genetic propensity to retain extra fat more easily or have a slower metabolic rate, making weight reduction more difficult. Furthermore, hormonal changes caused by aging or certain medical disorders might have an influence on metabolism and appetite regulation, affecting weight management attempts.

Understanding these individual distinctions is critical for developing a successful and lasting weight reduction plan for each person's specific goals and circumstances. Individuals can create a personalized strategy for weight loss that promotes success while minimizing hurdles by considering aspects such as personal preferences, lifestyle restrictions, and metabolic features.

Furthermore, the science of weight reduction highlights the significance of taking a complete strategy that includes not just food and exercise habits but also psychological, social, and environmental aspects. Stress management, mindfulness techniques, social support, and environmental adjustments can all help you lose weight successfully.

The science of weight reduction is broad and dynamic, encompassing biological, psychological, and environmental aspects. Individuals who grasp these basic concepts and individual characteristics may build successful and long-term methods for starting and maintaining a weight reduction program that improves general health and well-being.

Factors Affecting Weight Gain and Loss

Factors affecting weight gain and loss depend on a variety of factors impact weight control, each with its own function in the intricate interplay of energy balance, metabolism, and general health. Understanding these characteristics is critical for successfully starting a weight reduction regimen and achieving long-term outcomes.

First and foremost, eating habits and food choices have a substantial influence on weight gain and loss. A diet consisting of processed foods, refined sugars, and bad fats can lead to increased calorie consumption and weight gain.

Prioritizing complete, nutrient-dense meals like fruits, vegetables, lean meats, and whole grains, on the other hand, can help you lose weight by delivering important nutrients while keeping your calorie consumption under control. Furthermore, meal sizes and eating habits play an important role in weight management.

Eating thoughtfully, paying attention to hunger and fullness cues, and exercising portion control can all help you avoid overeating and lose weight.

Physical activity and exercise are both equally vital for weight control. Regular exercise not only burns calories, but it also improves metabolic health, builds lean muscle mass, and boosts general well-being. Incorporating aerobic activity, strength training, and flexibility exercises into your weekly regimen will help you lose and maintain weight effectively.

In addition to food and exercise, hormone modulation is essential for weight management. Hormones, including insulin, leptin, ghrelin, and cortisol, and thyroid hormones, affect hunger, metabolism, and fat storage. Variables such as nutrition, stress, sleep habits, and underlying medical disorders frequently impact these hormones, disrupting weight control and leading to weight gain or trouble decreasing weight.

Lifestyle factors such as stress, sleep quality, and socioeconomic position can all influence weight control. Chronic stress can cause emotional eating, alter hormone balance, and increase fat accumulation, whereas insufficient sleep can affect appetite-regulating hormones and metabolic processes, resulting in weight gain.

Genetic and metabolic variations can also have an impact on weight management. Some people may be genetically predisposed to retain extra fat more easily or have a slower metabolic rate, making weight reduction more difficult. Understanding these individual distinctions is critical for developing a successful and lasting weight reduction plan for each person's specific goals and circumstances.

Furthermore, environmental variables such as availability of healthy food alternatives, financial position, cultural influences, and societal standards have a substantial impact on weight control. Individuals living in food deserts, where fresh, nutritious foods are scarce, may struggle to maintain a balanced diet and control their weight. Similarly, cultural traditions and societal forces can shape food preferences, eating habits, and body image judgments, all of which have an impact on weight control practices.

Social support and the social environment around you heavily influence weight management. A supportive network of family, friends, or peers who encourage healthy behaviors and give accountability can significantly improve motivation and adherence to a weight reduction regimen.

In contrast, a lack of social support or exposure to unfavorable social factors can impede success and impair weight-loss efforts. A complex interaction of biological, psychological, social, environmental, and hereditary variables regulates weight gain and loss. Individuals may establish the groundwork for a successful weight reduction regimen that supports long-term and sustainable outcomes by thoroughly understanding and addressing these aspects. Starting a weight reduction journey entails not just adopting dietary and activity modifications but also taking into account the larger context of one's lifestyle, surroundings, and personal circumstances.

Individuals may embark on a road of improved health, well-being, and weight control by taking a holistic approach and committing to making good changes. Setting realistic goals setting realistic goals is the key to starting your weight-loss journey.

Starting a weight reduction journey might seem like venturing into unknown territory, full of enthusiasm, dedication, and even a trace of trepidation. As you lace up your sneakers and are ready to take the first step, it's critical to create realistic goals that will lead you to success. Picture this: You're standing at the foot of a mountain, looking up at the towering summit.

Your aim is to reach the peak, but you understand that it will not happen overnight. You recognize that it will take effort, persistence, and a number of minor milestones along the way.

Setting Realistic Goals

Setting realistic goals in your weight reduction journey is analogous to charting a course to the mountain top. It's about breaking down your ultimate objective into doable tasks that you can complete one at a time. It is about preparing yourself for success by understanding your starting place, accepting your limits, and appreciating your accomplishments along the way. So, what does it mean to have realistic goals? It entails creating specified, measurable, attainable, relevant, and time-bound targets, or SMART goals. Specific: Rather than loosely attempting to "lose weight," specify specifically what you intend to accomplish. Is there a set number of pounds? A dress size? Increased fitness levels? Measurable: Quantify your goals so that you can measure your progress.

Whether you're counting calories, charting exercises, or quantifying inches lost, having clear measurements can help you stay accountable and inspired.

Achievable: Be honest with yourself about what you can actually do. Set goals that are challenging yet achievable. Prefer making moderate and steady progress over attempting big changes that will not be sustained. Relevant: Your goals should be consistent with your overarching vision and principles. Consider why you want to reduce weight: for better health, more energy, or greater confidence.

Keep your "why" in mind when setting your goals. Set a time limit for yourself to work within. Whether it's a weekly, monthly, or quarterly objective, setting deadlines will help you feel more motivated and focused. Instead of declaring, "I want to lose 50 pounds," a SMART goal would be, "I will lose 1-2 pounds per week by following a balanced diet and exercising for 30 minutes, five days a week, for the next six months." Setting realistic objectives that are detailed, quantifiable, achievable, relevant, and time-bound prepares you for a successful weight reduction journey.

You're developing a road map that will guide you through the ups and downs while keeping you motivated and focused on your ultimate goal. As you begin your weight-loss journey, remember that setting realistic goals is more than just the numbers on the scale. It's also important to maintain a positive attitude and focus on small victories. Celebrate moments of increased energy, improved mood, better sleep, and greater strength and endurance.

Your approach to goal-setting must be flexible and adaptable. As you travel, you may encounter obstacles, setbacks, or unexpected changes in circumstances. Rather than viewing these challenges as failures, consider them opportunities for growth and learning.

Adjust your goals as needed, break them down into smaller steps, and continue forward with determination and resilience. Seek support and accountability from others who have similar goals or have been on weight-loss journeys. Joining a support group, working with a workout buddy, or seeking the advice of a health coach or nutritionist can all provide valuable encouragement, motivation, and guidance along the way. Setting realistic goals is the foundation for starting a successful weight-loss routine.

By adhering to the SMART criteria and focusing on both scale and non-scale victories, you can create a road map that will lead you to your ultimate goal of improved health and well-being. Stay committed, remain positive, and remember that every step forward, no matter how small, counts toward your goals.

Remember, Rome was not built in a day, nor will your weight-loss journey be. Embrace the process, celebrate your successes, big and small, and keep your sights set on the summit. With determination, perseverance, and SMART goals as your guide, you'll be well on your way to a healthier, happier you.

You have got this!

CHAPTER 2: BUILDING A FOUNDATION FOR SUCCESS

Success Building a foundation for success is the cornerstone of starting a weight-loss routine. Starting a weight reduction journey is similar to building a strong structure; it requires a solid foundation to ensure long-term success.

Before delving into the details of nutrition and exercise, it's critical to create the foundations for success. This foundation is built on three critical pillars: **analyzing existing behaviors and lifestyles, developing a healthy mentality, and creating a supportive environment.**

Assessing Current Habits and Lifestyle

Assessing current habits and lifestyles Assessing Current Habits and Lifestyles:

The First Step in Your Weight Loss Journey. Consider standing on the brink of huge, uncharted terrain, preparing to start on an exciting journey. This landscape depicts your weight-loss journey, which is full of discovery, development, and transformation. However, before embarking on this path, you must first assess your existing situation: your habits, lifestyle, and choices. Assessing your present habits and lifestyle is akin to casting a light into the darkest corners of your life, revealing the patterns and behaviors that have molded your connection with food, exercise, and general well-being. It's about exposing the layers of your daily routine, from the foods you consume to the activities you do, and understanding how they affect your present state of health.

Begin by examining your eating habits with an inquisitive eye. What meals do you usually reach for during the day? Do you find yourself grabbing for sugary foods when you're anxious or munching mindlessly while watching TV? Take note of your portion amounts, meal scheduling, and nutritional balance in your diet. Are you feeding your body nutritious foods that promote health and vitality, or are you depending on processed, calorie-laden meals that leave you feeling lethargic and unsatisfied? Next, assess your degree of physical activity.

How often do you move your body during the day? Do you exercise regularly, or do you live a sedentary lifestyle? Consider the activities you like and how to incorporate them into your everyday routine. Perhaps it's a brisk morning stroll, an evening yoga session, or a weekend dancing class with pals.

Find methods to include movement in your daily routine in a way that feels natural and joyful. Evaluate both your sleep patterns and quality. How many hours of sleep do you get every night? Do you follow a consistent nighttime ritual that promotes calm and peaceful sleep, or do you find yourself browsing through your phone late at night? Recognize the significance of excellent sleep in maintaining general health and weight control, and prioritize setting a sleep environment and habit that promote restorative sleep.

Also, think about your stress levels and coping techniques. How do you handle stress in your life? Do you seek consolation via food, or do you have healthy coping methods in place? Take notice of the pressures in your life and look into alternate ways to manage them, such as meditation, deep breathing exercises, or participating in hobbies and activities that you like. As you continue to evaluate your habits and lifestyle, consider the emotional and psychological components of your relationship with food and exercise.

Consider your reasons for trying to reduce weight and how your emotions could impact your eating habits. Are you eating because you are hungry, or do you eat to relieve stress, boredom, or other emotions? Recognizing and treating emotional eating behaviors is critical to building a better relationship with food and achieving long-term weight reduction success.

Furthermore, analyze how your social and environmental surroundings influence your behaviors and lifestyle. Do your friends and family support your health objectives, or do they encourage harmful habits? How does your work environment or social circle affect your eating habits and physical activity levels? Identifying possible triggers or hurdles in your social and environmental context will help you establish successful techniques for navigating them and staying on track with your weight reduction goals.

Understanding your sleep patterns and how they affect Weight control is another critical component of examining your habits and lifestyle. Research has linked poor sleep quality and inadequate sleep duration to weight gain and an increased risk of obesity.

Examine your sleep hygiene behaviors, including your evening ritual, sleeping environment, and use of electronic devices before bedtime. Making minor changes to enhance your sleep quality can have a huge impact on your overall health and weight reduction attempts.

 Finally, think about your general health and any underlying medical concerns that might affect your weight-reduction quest. Consult a healthcare expert to assess your present health, address any medical issues or problems, and verify that your weight reduction objectives are compatible with your general health and well-being.

Taking a holistic approach to examining your behaviors and lifestyle provides useful insights into the elements driving your weight management attempts. With this knowledge, you may create a tailored weight reduction plan that matches your specific requirements, difficulties, and goals. Remember, this journey is about more than simply losing weight; it's about living a healthier, happier life for yourself, one step at a time.

Assessing your present habits and lifestyle with honesty and inquiry can provide significant insights into the elements that have led to your current state of health and well-being. Armed with this knowledge, you can start identifying areas for improvement and laying the framework for a weight loss regimen personalized to your own requirements and circumstances. So, take a deep breath, enjoy this moment of self-reflection, and prepare to begin on the adventure of a lifetime—your path to a better, happier you.

Establishing a Healthy Mindset

Developing a Healthy Mindset: Building a solid foundation for success also entails building a positive mentality that promotes drive, resilience, and self-compassion.

Adopting a good attitude and viewing weight reduction as a journey rather than a destination might help you overcome obstacles and stay focused on your objectives. Set reasonable expectations and accept the idea of progress over perfection. Understand that setbacks and challenges are unavoidable, but they also present chances for development and learning. Approach your weight reduction journey with curiosity, openness, and a willingness to try out new tactics to see what works best for you. Practice self-compassion and gentleness toward oneself, especially during times of adversity or setbacks.

Instead of participating in negative self-talk or self-criticism, treat yourself with the same kindness and compassion that you would show a friend facing comparable circumstances.

The Key to Beginning Your Weight Loss Journey

Starting a weight-reduction journey entails not only altering your physical habits but also improving your thinking. Building a healthy mentality is critical for long-term success because it influences your attitudes, beliefs, and habits around diet, exercise, and general well-being. Here's how you may develop a healthy mentality to launch your weight reduction regimen:

1. **Shift Your Perspective:** Begin by viewing weight reduction as a journey of self-discovery and personal progress rather than a fast cure or temporary answer. Accept the concept that this journey is about more than simply losing weight; it's about developing a better, happier lifestyle that improves your total well-being.

2. **Practice self-compassion:** Be nice and patient with yourself during your weight reduction journey. Understand that failures and hurdles are unavoidable and do not define your worth or success. Treat yourself with the same care

and understanding that you would extend to a friend facing comparable circumstances.

3. **Focus on Progress, Not Perfection:** Let go of the idea of perfection and instead applaud every progress, no matter how minor. Recognize and appreciate every positive step you take toward your objectives, whether it's eating healthier, adhering to an exercise plan, or practicing self-care.

4. **Set realistic expectations:** Be realistic about your goals and the time frame in which you can attain them. Set tough but realistic goals, and then break them down into smaller, more doable steps. Avoid comparing yourself to others and concentrate on your own success and development.

5. **Develop a Growth Mindset:** Embrace the belief that hard work, practice, and patience can improve your talents and intelligence. View challenges and failures as chances for learning and progress rather than impassable hurdles.

6. **Practice Mindfulness:** Integrate mindfulness techniques into your everyday routine to increase awareness and self-compassion. Savor each bite, listen to your body's hunger and fullness cues, and focus on the sensations and flavors

of your meal. In addition, use mindfulness meditation or deep breathing techniques to relieve stress and increase emotional well-being.

7. **Focus on non-scale successes:** Instead of focusing on the number on the scale, celebrate non-scale successes—accomplishments that go beyond weight reduction. This might include increases in energy, mood, sleep quality, physical fitness, and general well-being.

8. **Surround Yourself with Positivity:** Surround yourself with positive influences that can help you achieve your goals and improve your spirits. Seek out friends, relatives, or online groups that will encourage and inspire you on your path. Surround yourself with positive messages, affirmations, and reminders of your accomplishments and potential.

9. **Embrace Flexibility and Adaptability:** Accept that your weight reduction journey may not always go as planned. Be willing to change your objectives and techniques as necessary based on your progress, preferences, and changing circumstances. Flexibility and

adaptation are essential for handling the highs and lows of your trip with resilience and determination.

10. **Practice Gratitude:** Develop a grateful mentality by concentrating on the good things in your life and path. Take time each day to focus on what you are grateful for, whether it is the support of loved ones, the chance to fuel your body with nutritious food, or the capacity to move and exercise. Practicing thankfulness may help you alter your viewpoint and thinking toward abundance and optimism, allowing you to handle obstacles with grace and appreciation.

11. **Challenge Negative Ideas:** Recognize any negative ideas or beliefs that may be preventing you from achieving your goals. Challenge these ideas by challenging their validity and reframing them in a more positive and powerful way. Replace self-critical thoughts with affirmations and phrases that encourage and urge you to continue going forward.

12. **Prioritize Long-Term Health:** Move your attention away from short-term weight loss objectives and toward long-term health and well-being. Rather than focusing on a

certain number on the scale, prioritize habits and behaviors that promote overall health, energy, and longevity. Accept lifestyle adjustments that promote your physical, mental, and emotional well-being, recognizing that long-term weight loss is a natural outcome of a healthy lifestyle.

13. **Prioritize Self-Care:** Make self-care a priority in your weight reduction journey by dedicating time to your physical, mental, and emotional well-being. Engage in things that provide you joy, relaxation, and contentment, such as reading a book, having a bubble bath, spending time in nature, or pursuing a hobby you like. Prioritizing self-care replenishes your energy and resilience, making it simpler to stay focused on your goals.

14. **Celebrate Your Development:** Take the time to recognize and celebrate your accomplishments and development along the way. Celebrate every milestone, no matter how minor, and use these moments to strengthen your devotion to your goals. Recognize the effort and commitment you've put into your trip, and be proud of your accomplishments.

Establishing a healthy mentality prepares you for success in your weight-reduction quest. Cultivating self-compassion, concentrating on progress, practicing mindfulness, and surrounding yourself with positivity are all critical components of a mentality that will help you achieve your objectives and generate long-term change in your life. Remember that your mentality is a powerful instrument that can create your reality, so build a mindset that promotes growth, resilience, and well-being as you begin on this transforming path.

Creating a Support System

Laying a solid foundation for success entails providing a supportive atmosphere that promotes healthy habits and behaviors. Surround yourself with individuals who share your goals and inspire you. Share your goals with friends, family, or coworkers who may offer encouragement, accountability, and practical help.

Make changes to your physical surroundings to encourage healthy habits. Stock your kitchen with healthy items and limit the availability of enticing, unhealthy snacks. Create a specific training area at home or join a facility that meets your fitness objectives and interests.

 Additionally, look for services and tools that can help you lose weight, such as meal planning apps, fitness trackers, online groups, or professional advice from a certified dietitian, personal trainer, or health coach.

Divide your goals into smaller, more manageable tasks that you can track and measure along the way. This will give you a sense of accomplishment and momentum, keeping you motivated and focused on your goals.

In addition, try implementing self-care techniques into your daily routine to improve your overall health. Prioritize activities that encourage relaxation, stress reduction, and mental clarity, such as yoga, meditation, writing, or spending time outside. Taking care of your mental and emotional health is essential for staying motivated and resilient on your weight-reduction journey.

Educate yourself on diet, exercise, and good living practices so that you may make educated decisions. Learn about the nutritional value of various foods, how to read food labels, and meal planning and preparation tips. Similarly, learn about different types of exercise, their advantages, and how to properly incorporate them into your daily routine.

As you lay the groundwork for success, remember to be patient and give yourself grace. Sustainable weight reduction requires patience, consistency, and perseverance. Focus on progress rather than perfection, and savor every tiny triumph along the way.

Nurturing your path to weight loss success

Starting a weight reduction journey may be both exciting and intimidating, but having a supportive network in place can greatly increase your chances of success. Creating a strong support system is critical for offering encouragement, inspiration, and accountability as you negotiate the obstacles and successes of beginning a weight reduction program.

The first step in developing a support system is to identify people in your life who are truly interested in your well-being and weight reduction objectives. These might include family members, friends, coworkers, or even online groups of people who have similar health goals. Look for people who are supportive, empathetic, and nonjudgmental, and who will encourage you as you go on your journey.

Once you've identified your supporters, tell them about your weight reduction objectives and ask for their aid in reaching them. Share your motives, problems, and success tactics, and be open about the level of help you require from them. Whether it's accompanying you for workouts, making healthy meals together, or delivering words of encouragement during difficult times, having a supportive network may be extremely beneficial in sticking to your objectives.

In addition to getting support from friends and family, you should consider working with a professional who can provide expert direction and accountability on your weight reduction journey. This might include a licensed nutritionist, personal trainer, or health coach who can provide tailored suggestions, track your progress, and offer encouragement and support along the way.

Joining health and wellness-focused groups or organizations can also help you discover the power of community. Connecting with people who share similar goals, whether through a local fitness class, a running club, or an online support group, may bring a sense of camaraderie as well as accountability. Surrounding yourself with others who are equally devoted to improving their health may inspire and drive you to stick with your weight reduction plan.

Beyond asking for help from others, don't overlook the need for self-care in developing your support system. Prioritize activities that improve your physical, mental, and emotional well-being, such as obtaining adequate sleep, practicing good stress management, and engaging in enjoyable and relaxing hobbies. Taking care of yourself not only helps you stay dedicated to your weight reduction objectives, but it also provides a good example for those in your support system.

Furthermore, developing a support system goes beyond the people in your life. It also entails building a supportive atmosphere that encourages your weight reduction objectives and promotes healthy habits. This may entail making adjustments to your physical environment, such as having nutritious snacks on hand, creating a separate workout area at home, or eliminating enticing, unhealthy meals from your living space.

In addition, consider using technology to improve your support system. There are several applications and online tools available to help you track your progress, interact with others going through similar experiences, and access essential resources and information. Whether it's a fitness app to track your exercises, a meal planning tool to simplify healthy eating, or an online group for accountability and support, technology may be a valuable partner in your weight loss journey.

Furthermore, do not overlook the significance of commemorating milestones and triumphs along the path. Recognize and reward yourself for your accomplishments, whether they be hitting a certain weight milestone, accomplishing a new exercise goal, or continuously adhering to your healthy habits. Celebrating your accomplishments promotes healthy habits and encourages you to keep moving forward on your quest.

Finally, remember that nurturing and maintaining a support system is an ongoing process. Stay in touch with your supporters, talk freely about your needs and concerns, and be proactive in requesting assistance when necessary.

Cultivating a solid support system requires time and work, but the rewards, such as improved motivation, accountability, and resilience, are well worth it.

Developing a support system is an essential part of starting a weight reduction regimen and ensuring long-lasting success. By surrounding yourself with supportive people, seeking professional advice, connecting with like-minded communities, and prioritizing self-care, you can create a strong network of support that will help you overcome obstacles, stay motivated, and achieve your weight-loss goals with confidence and resilience.

Remember that you do not have to go through this path alone; with the help of others, you may improve your health and well-being significantly.

Let's look at how to set up a support system while starting a weight reduction routine:

Consider Jane, who has decided to start a weight-loss journey to better her health and well-being. Jane understands that having a supportive network will be critical to keeping her motivated and accountable during her journey. Here's how she sets up her support system:

1. Family Support: Jane tells her spouse and children about her weight reduction objectives, explaining why she wants to make better choices and how they can help her. They vow to support her in developing healthy eating habits as a family, such as cooking nutritious meals together and paying attention to portion sizes. Her husband also offers to take on extra domestic tasks so Sarah may concentrate on her exercises.

2. Friend Accountability: Jane contacts a close friend who has indicated interest in improving her health. They decide to be accountability partners, communicating on a regular basis to discuss progress, support one another, and celebrate wins. They want to meet for weekly walks or workouts to keep each other motivated and accountable.

3. Professional assistance: Jane makes an appointment with a certified dietitian to receive specific dietary advice and assistance. The nutritionist assists Sarah in developing a balanced meal plan that is consistent with her weight reduction objectives, as well as practical ways for dealing with typical issues like desire management and dining out.

Jane also hires a personal trainer, who creates an exercise regimen according to her fitness level and goals.

4. Online Community Support: Jane joins an online weight loss community to connect with others who are on a similar journey. She takes part in group challenges, provides progress updates, and receives support and encouragement from other members. Jane feels motivated to stick to her healthy habits because of the sense of camaraderie and responsibility that the community provides.

5. Self-Care and Celebration: Throughout her journey, Jane prioritizes self-care activities to manage stress and refuel her energy. She meditates, takes calming baths, and spends quality time with her loved ones. Jane also celebrates accomplishments along the way, such as meeting a specific weight reduction goal or finishing a difficult activity. She gives herself non-food rewards, such as a spa day or new training gear, to recognize her hard work and devotion.

Sarah prepares herself for weight reduction success by developing a complete support system that includes family support, friend accountability, professional assistance, online community support, and self-care routines. Sarah feels inspired and driven to overcome difficulties and reach her weight reduction objectives with confidence and commitment, thanks to her support system's encouragement, accountability, and resources.

I'm starting my weight loss journey with a solid support system! Family, friends, professionals, and internet groups are rooting for me every step of the way. Let us accomplish this! #WeightLossSupport

Chapter 3: Nutrition Essentials

The Foundation of a Successful Weight Loss Routine Starting a weight loss routine involves more than just increasing physical activity; it requires a fundamental shift in your approach to nutrition. Nutrition plays a central role in weight management, providing your body with the essential nutrients it needs while supporting your overall health and well-being.

Here are the key nutrition essentials to consider when starting a weight loss routine:

1. **Balanced Diet:** Adopting a balanced diet is essential for providing your body with the nutrients it needs to thrive while promoting weight loss. Aim to include a variety of nutrient-dense foods from all food groups, including fruits, vegetables, whole grains, lean proteins, and healthy fats. Focus on incorporating whole, minimally processed foods that are rich in vitamins, minerals, fiber, and antioxidants.

Let's break it down.

Balanced Diet: A balanced diet is the cornerstone of a successful weight loss routine. It involves consuming a variety of foods from all food groups to ensure your body receives the essential nutrients it needs for optimal health and function. This includes fruits and vegetables, which provide essential vitamins, minerals, fiber, and antioxidants that support overall health and aid in weight management. Aim to fill half of your plate with colorful fruits and vegetables at each meal.

Whole Grains: Choose whole grains such as brown rice, quinoa, oats, and whole wheat bread over refined grains. Whole grains are rich in fiber, which helps promote satiety and digestive health.

Lean Proteins: Incorporate lean protein sources such as chicken, turkey, fish, tofu, beans, lentils, and Greek yogurt into your meals. Protein helps build and repair tissues, supports muscle growth, and promotes feelings of fullness.

Healthy Fats: Include sources of healthy fats such as avocados, nuts, seeds, olive oil, and fatty fish like salmon and sardines. Healthy fats provide energy, support brain health, and aid in the absorption of fat-soluble vitamins.

2. **Portion Control:** Paying attention to portion sizes is crucial for managing calorie intake and promoting weight loss. Be mindful of serving sizes and avoid oversized portions, especially when dining out or consuming packaged foods. Using smaller plates, measuring portions, and practicing mindful eating can help you better control portion sizes and prevent overeating. Tips for practicing portion control include using smaller plates and bowls to help control portion sizes. Measuring or weighing food portions, especially calorie-dense foods like nuts, oils, and grains, Be mindful of portion sizes when dining out or eating packaged foods, as restaurant portions and packaged servings are often larger than necessary.

3. **Macronutrient Balance:** Balancing your intake of macronutrients—carbohydrates, protein, and fat—is key for supporting weight loss and overall health. Aim to include a balance of all three macronutrients in each meal and snack to promote satiety, stabilize blood sugar levels, and maintain energy levels throughout the day.

Focus on incorporating high-quality sources of carbohydrates, lean proteins, and healthy fats into your diet. Each macronutrient plays a specific role in your body and should be included in your diet in appropriate proportions.

Carbohydrates: Choose complex carbohydrates such as whole grains, fruits, and vegetables, which provide sustained energy and fiber for digestive health. Protein: Incorporate lean protein sources into each meal to support muscle growth, repair, and satiety.

 Fat: Include sources of healthy fats in your diet to support hormone production, brain health, and the absorption of fat-soluble vitamins.

4. **Hydration:** Staying hydrated is essential for supporting overall health and facilitating weight loss. Drinking an adequate amount of water throughout the day helps regulate appetite, boost metabolism, and support proper digestion and nutrient absorption. Aim to drink at least eight glasses of water per day, and consider incorporating hydrating foods such as fruits and vegetables into your diet.

 5. **Mindful Eating:** Practicing mindful eating involves paying attention to your body's hunger and fullness cues, as

well as your emotions and surroundings, while eating. Slow down and savor each bite, chew your food thoroughly, and listen to your body's signals of hunger and fullness. Avoid distractions such as screens or multitasking while eating, as they can lead to mindless overeating. Tips for practicing mindful eating include eating slowly and savoring each bite.

Paying attention to hunger and fullness cues. Minimizing distractions such as screens or multitasking while eating. Listening to your body's signals and stopping when you feel satisfied, rather than overly full.

6. **Meal Planning and Preparation:** Planning and preparing meals in advance can help you make healthier choices and avoid impulsive or unhealthy food choices. Take time to plan your meals and snacks for the week, create a grocery list, and batch cook or prep ingredients ahead of time. Having nutritious meals and snacks readily available can make it easier to stick to your weight-loss goals and resist temptation. Tips for meal planning and preparation include: planning your meals and snacks for the week ahead of time.

Creating a grocery list based on your meal plan will ensure you have all the ingredients you need. Batch cooking or prepping ingredients in advance to save time during the week. Packing healthy snacks and meals to take with you when you're on the go.

7. **Flexibility and Moderation:** While it's important to prioritize nutrient-dense foods, it's also essential to allow for flexibility and moderation in your diet. Incorporate your favorite foods in moderation, practice portion control, and enjoy treats occasionally without guilt or restriction. Strive for balance and sustainability in your eating habits, rather than aiming for perfection or strict adherence to a specific diet. Tips for practicing flexibility and moderation include incorporating your favorite foods into your diet in moderation.

Practicing portion control and mindful eating when indulging in treats. Avoiding labeling foods as "good" or "bad" and instead focusing on balance and moderation. Remember that occasional indulgences are part of a healthy, balanced lifestyle. Focusing on nutrition essentials is crucial for starting a successful weight-loss routine. By adopting a balanced diet, practicing portion control, balancing macronutrients, staying hydrated, practicing mindful eating, meal planning and preparation, and allowing for flexibility and moderation, you can lay the foundation for a sustainable and effective weight loss journey.

Remember, making gradual, sustainable changes to your eating habits is key to achieving long-term success and maintaining a healthy weight for life.

Understanding Macronutrients and Micronutrients

The fascinating world of macronutrients and micronutrients—the essential building blocks of a healthy diet and the key to kick starting your weight loss routine! Imagine your body as a high-performance machine, fueled by a precise combination of nutrients to keep it running smoothly. Macronutrients are like the fuel that powers your engine, while micronutrients are the tiny, yet powerful, tools that keep everything running in tip-top shape.

Let's talk about macronutrients—the big three: carbohydrates, proteins, and fats. Carbs are your body's main source of energy and are found in delicious foods like whole grains, fruits, and vegetables.

They're like the high-octane fuel that gives you the energy to crush your workouts and power through your day. Next, we have proteins—the muscle builders and repairers. Proteins, found in foods like lean meats, poultry, fish, beans, and tofu, are essential for building and repairing muscles, keeping you strong and lean as you shed those extra pounds. And let's not forget about fats—the misunderstood superheroes of your diet. Healthy fats, like those found in avocados, nuts, seeds, and fatty fish, are essential for brain health, hormone production, and keeping you feeling full and satisfied. Now, onto micronutrients—the unsung heroes of nutrition. While they may be small in size, micronutrients pack a powerful punch when it comes to supporting your overall health and weight loss goals.

These include vitamins, minerals, and antioxidants found in a colorful array of fruits, vegetables, nuts, seeds, and whole grains. Vitamins and minerals act as co-factors in hundreds of metabolic processes in your body, from energy production to immune function and everything in between. Antioxidants, on the other hand, help fight off oxidative stress and inflammation, keeping your cells healthy and your body functioning at its best. But here's the kicker: while macronutrients provide the energy your body needs to function, it's the micronutrients that provide the essential tools for optimal health and weight loss success. So, while you're focusing on counting macros and watching your calories, don't forget to load up on those colorful fruits and veggies to ensure you're getting all the essential micronutrients your body needs to thrive.

The role of macronutrients and micronutrients is crucial for kick starting your weight loss routine. By fueling your body with the right balance of carbs, proteins, and fats, along with a rainbow of colorful fruits and veggies rich in essential vitamins, minerals, and antioxidants, you'll set yourself up for success on your weight loss journey. So, go ahead and fill your plate with nutrient-dense foods, and watch as your body transforms into the lean, mean, fat-burning machine you've always dreamed of.

Developing a Balanced Meal Plan

Your Blueprint for Weight Loss Success Starting a weight loss routine involves more than just exercising; it requires a holistic approach that includes creating a balanced meal plan to support your goals. A well-designed meal plan ensures that you're nourishing your body with the right combination of nutrients while creating a sustainable eating pattern that promotes weight loss.

Here's how to develop a balanced meal plan to kick start your weight loss journey:

1. **Assess Your Current Eating Habits:** Before creating a meal plan, take some time to assess your current eating habits. Keep a food diary for a few days to track what and when you eat, as well as your portion sizes. This will help you identify any patterns or areas where you may need to make changes to support your weight-loss goals.

2. **Set realistic goals:** Determine your weight loss goals and establish a realistic timeline for achieving them. Aim for gradual, sustainable weight loss of 1-2 pounds per week, which is considered safe and achievable for most

people. Keep in mind that weight loss is not just about the number on the scale but also about improving your overall health and well-being.

3. Calculate Your Calorie Needs: To lose weight, you need to create a calorie deficit by consuming fewer calories than your body needs to maintain its current weight. Use an online calculator or consult with a nutritionist to estimate your daily calorie needs based on factors such as your age, gender, weight, height, activity level, and weight loss goals.

4. Choose Nutrient-Dense Foods: Focus on incorporating nutrient-dense foods into your meal plan, including fruits, vegetables, lean proteins, whole grains, and healthy fats. These foods are rich in vitamins, minerals, fiber, and antioxidants, which are essential for supporting overall health and weight loss. Aim to fill half of your plate with colorful fruits and vegetables at each meal.

5. Balance Your Macronutrients: Ensure that your meal plan includes a balance of macronutrients—carbohydrates, proteins, and fats—to support your energy needs, muscle growth, and satiety. Aim to include a source of lean protein, healthy fats, and complex carbohydrates in each meal to create a balanced and satisfying plate.

6. Plan Your Meals and Snacks: Once you have a good understanding of your calorie needs and nutrient requirements, start planning your meals and snacks for the week ahead. Consider your schedule, preferences, and cooking abilities when creating your meal plan, and aim for variety and balance to keep things interesting and enjoyable.

7. Practice Portion Control: Be mindful of portion sizes and practice portion control to avoid overeating and support your weight loss goals. Use measuring cups, spoons, or a food scale to portion out your food, especially calorie-dense foods like nuts, oils, and grains. Fill your plate with appropriate portions of each food group to ensure a balanced and satisfying meal.

8. Include Healthy Snacks: Plan for healthy snacks to keep you satisfied between meals and prevent overeating. Choose nutrient-dense snacks such as fresh fruit, Greek yogurt, nuts, seeds, whole grain crackers with hummus, or vegetable sticks with guacamole. Keep portion sizes in check and avoid mindless snacking by portioning out snacks in advance.

9. Stay Hydrated: Don't forget to include plenty of fluids in your meal plan to stay hydrated throughout the day. Aim to drink at least eight glasses of water per day and include hydrating beverages such as herbal tea, infused water, or sparkling water with lemon or cucumber slices. Limit sugary drinks and alcohol, which can add extra calories and hinder weight-loss efforts.

10. Be Flexible and Adjust as Needed: Remember that your meal plan is a flexible guide, not a rigid set of rules. Be open to adjusting your plan based on your progress, preferences, and changing circumstances. Listen to your body's hunger and fullness cues and make adjustments as needed to ensure you're meeting your nutritional needs while staying on track with your weight loss goals.

By following these steps and developing a balanced meal plan tailored to your needs and preferences, you'll set yourself up for success on your weight-loss journey.

A balanced meal plan ensures that you're nourishing your body with the right combination of nutrients while creating a sustainable eating pattern that supports your weight loss goals and promotes overall health and well-being.

Remember to stay consistent, be mindful of your portion sizes, and celebrate your progress along the way.

Incorporating Superfoods and Nutrient-Dense Foods

Fueling Your Weight Loss Journey with Power-Packed Nutrition When embarking on a weight loss journey, incorporating superfoods and nutrient-dense foods into your diet can be a game-changer. These powerhouse foods are rich in essential vitamins, minerals, antioxidants, and other beneficial nutrients that support overall health and well-being while promoting weight loss.

Let's explore how to incorporate these nutrient-packed options into your daily meals to kick-start your weight loss routine:

1. Leafy Greens: Leafy greens such as spinach, kale, Swiss chard, and collard greens are nutritional powerhouses packed with vitamins, minerals, and antioxidants. Incorporating leafy greens into your meals adds volume and fiber, helping you feel full and satisfied while keeping calorie intake in check. Try adding a handful of spinach to your morning smoothie, tossing kale into salads, or sautéing Swiss chard as a nutritious side dish.

2. Berries: Berries such as blueberries, strawberries, raspberries, and blackberries are low in calories but high in fiber, vitamins, and antioxidants. Adding berries to your meals and snacks provides a burst of flavor and sweetness without added sugars, making them a perfect choice for satisfying cravings while supporting weight loss. Enjoy berries on their own as a refreshing snack, or add them to oatmeal, yogurt, or salads for a delicious and nutritious boost.

3. Lean Proteins: Incorporating lean proteins such as chicken breast, turkey, fish, tofu, tempeh, and legumes into your meals supports muscle growth, repair, and satiety while keeping calorie intake in check. Opt for lean cuts of meat, remove visible fat, and choose cooking methods such as grilling, baking, or steaming to keep added fats to a minimum. Include a source of lean protein in each meal to promote fullness and support your weight-loss goals.

4. Whole Grains: Whole grains such as quinoa, brown rice, oats, barley, and farro are rich in fiber, vitamins, minerals, and antioxidants, making them a nutritious addition to your weight loss routine. Incorporating whole grains into your meals provides sustained energy, promotes digestive health, and helps keep you feeling full and satisfied. Swap refined grains for whole grains in dishes like salads, stir-fries, soups, and grain bowls to boost nutritional content and support weight loss.

5. Healthy Fats: Incorporating healthy fats such as avocados, nuts, seeds, olive oil, and fatty fish into your meals provides essential fatty acids, vitamins, and antioxidants that support heart health, brain function, and overall well-being. While fats are calorie-dense, they also help promote satiety and keep you feeling full and satisfied between meals. Add a slice of avocado to your toast, sprinkle nuts and seeds on salads, or drizzle olive oil over roasted vegetables to incorporate healthy fats into your diet.

6. Greek Yogurt: Greek yogurt is a nutrient-dense food rich in protein, calcium, probiotics, and essential vitamins and minerals. Incorporating Greek yogurt into your meals and snacks provides a creamy and satisfying option that supports muscle growth, bone health, and digestive function. Incorporate Greek yogurt into your breakfast by topping it with fruit and granola, or use it as a creamy base for smoothies, dips, and sauces.

7. Colorful vegetables like bell peppers, carrots, tomatoes, broccoli, and sweet potatoes contain vitamins, minerals, antioxidants, and fiber that promote overall health and aid in weight loss. Incorporating a variety of colorful vegetables into your meals adds flavor, texture, and nutritional value while keeping calorie intake in check. Roast vegetables as a flavorful side dish, add them to stir-fries, salads, or soups, or enjoy them raw with hummus or yogurt-based dips.

8. Legumes: Legumes such as beans, lentils, chickpeas, and peas are nutrient-dense plant-based sources of protein, fiber, vitamins, and minerals that support weight loss and overall health. Incorporating legumes into your meals adds bulk, texture, and nutritional value while promoting satiety and supporting digestive health. Add beans to soups, stews, salads, or grain bowls, or enjoy them as a protein-rich side dish or main course.

9. Chia Seeds: Chia seeds are tiny but mighty superfoods packed with fiber, protein, omega-3 fatty acids, and various vitamins and minerals. Incorporating chia seeds into your meals and snacks adds a nutritional boost and helps promote feelings of fullness and satiety. Sprinkle chia seeds on top of yogurt or oatmeal, add them to smoothies, or use them as a thickening agent in homemade puddings or overnight oats for a nutritious and satisfying treat.

10. Cruciferous Vegetables: Cruciferous vegetables such as broccoli, cauliflower, Brussels sprouts, and cabbage are nutritional powerhouses rich in vitamins, minerals, and antioxidants. Incorporating cruciferous vegetables into your meals provides numerous health benefits, including supporting detoxification, promoting heart health, and aiding in weight loss. Enjoy cruciferous vegetables roasted, steamed, or sautéed as a flavorful side dish, or add them to salads, stir-fries, or soups for a nutritious and delicious boost.

11. **Flaxseeds:** Flaxseeds are another nutrient-dense superfood rich in fiber, omega-3 fatty acids, and lignans, which have antioxidant properties. Incorporating flaxseeds into your diet supports digestive health, heart health, and overall well-being. For a nutritional boost, add ground flaxseeds to smoothies, oatmeal, yogurt, or baked goods, and use whole flaxseeds as a topping for salads or in homemade granola or energy bars.

12. Green tea, a popular beverage rich in antioxidants, particularly catechism, has been shown to support weight loss and metabolic health. Incorporating green tea into your daily routine provides hydration and antioxidant benefits while supporting your weight-loss goals. Enjoy green tea as a refreshing beverage on its own, or add it to smoothies or homemade iced tea for a flavorful and nutritious boost.

13. Quinoa: Quinoa is a versatile and nutrient-dense whole grain rich in protein, fiber, vitamins, and minerals. Incorporating quinoa into your meals provides sustained energy, promotes satiety, and supports overall health and well-being. Use quinoa as a base for salads, grain bowls, or stir-fries, or enjoy it as a side dish or main course in place of rice or pasta for a nutritious and satisfying meal.

14. Walnuts: Walnuts are nutrient-dense nuts rich in omega-3 fatty acids, antioxidants, and various vitamins and minerals. Incorporating walnuts into your diet supports heart health, brain function, and overall well-being. Enjoy walnuts as a snack on their own, add them to salads, oatmeal, or yogurt, or use them as a crunchy topping for baked goods or savory dishes for a nutritious and delicious boost.

15. Sweet Potatoes: Sweet potatoes are nutrient-dense root vegetables rich in fiber, vitamins, minerals, and antioxidants. Incorporating sweet potatoes into your meals provides sustained energy, promotes digestive health, and supports overall well-being. Enjoy sweet potatoes roasted, baked, mashed, or grilled as a flavorful side dish or main course, or add them to salads, soups, or stews for a nutritious and satisfying meal. Incorporating superfoods and nutrient-dense foods into your diet is a powerful strategy for fueling your weight-loss journey with power-packed nutrition. By including a variety of leafy greens, berries, lean proteins, whole grains, healthy fats, Greek yogurt, colorful vegetables, and legumes in your meals and snacks, you'll nourish your body with essential nutrients while supporting your weight-loss goals.

Experiment with different recipes, flavors, and textures to keep your meals exciting and satisfying, and enjoy the delicious journey to a healthier, happier you!

CHAPTER 4: EXERCISE AND PHYSICAL ACTIVITY

Key Components of a Successful Weight Loss Routine

When it comes to losing weight, integrating exercise and physical activity is critical for burning calories, developing muscle, improving cardiovascular health, and increasing overall well-being.

Let's go more into the significance of exercise and physical activity in your weight reduction routine:

1. **Types of Exercises:** There are different sorts of exercise, each with its own benefits for weight reduction and overall health.

   - **Cardiovascular Exercise:** Cardiovascular exercise, also known as aerobic exercise, is any activity that raises your heart rate and increases your breathing rate, such as walking, running, cycling, swimming, dancing, or utilizing cardio devices like treadmills or ellipticals.

Cardiovascular activity burns calories, improves cardiovascular health, and contributes to the calorie deficit required for weight loss. Strength - **Training:** Strength training, also known as resistance training or weightlifting, is employing resistance (dumbbells, resistance bands, or your own body weight) to increase muscle strength and endurance. Strength exercise promotes lean muscle growth, increases metabolism, and improves body composition by lowering body fat percentage.

- **Flexibility and Mobility Exercises:** Yoga, Pilates, stretching, and mobility drills can help improve joint flexibility, range of motion, and posture. Incorporating flexibility exercises into your program can help avoid injuries, minimize muscle soreness, and improve overall movement quality.

2. **Frequency, duration, and intensity:** To optimize the effects of exercise for weight reduction, you should evaluate the frequency, length, and intensity of your exercises. Frequency: Aim to complete at

least 150 minutes of moderate-intensity aerobic activity or 75 minutes of vigorous-intensity aerobic exercise each week, spaced out over multiple days. Incorporate strength training workouts targeting key muscle groups at least twice each week.

3. **Duration:** Cardiovascular workouts should last 20 to 60 minutes per session, depending on your fitness level and objectives.

   Strength training sessions typically take 30 to 60 minutes, including warm-up and cool-down periods.

4. **Intensity:** The intensity of your exercises may be quantified in a variety of ways, including heart rate, subjective effort, and metabolic equivalents (METs). During cardiovascular exercise, aim for a moderate-to-strong effort level that will push you yet allow you to sustain a conversation. When strength training, choose weights that allow you to accomplish 8 to 12 repetitions with perfect technique before tiring.

5. **Integrating Physical Activity into Daily Life:** In addition to regular exercise sessions, adding physical activity to your daily life will enhance

calorie expenditure and support your weight reduction attempts. Instead of driving, walk or bike short distances or run errands. Use the stairs instead of the elevator.

If you work in a sedentary environment, stand up and walk about often. Pursue active activities such as gardening, dancing, or athletics. Schedule activity breaks throughout the day to stretch or go for a brief stroll.

6. **Progress and Variety:** To keep making progress and avoiding plateaus in your weight reduction journey, add progression and variation to your workout program.

7. **Progression:** As your fitness improves, gradually increase the intensity, length, and frequency of your workouts. This might include lifting heavier weights during strength training, including intervals or inclinations into aerobic routines, or attempting more difficult types of activities.

8. **Variety:** Use a variety of exercises, activities, and training forms to keep your program interesting and prevent boredom. This might involve attempting

new types of aerobic workouts, changing up your strength training program, or discovering new fitness classes or hobbies.

9. **Rest and recovery:** Finally, don't underestimate the value of rest and recuperation in your weight reduction efforts. Schedule one to two rest days per week to allow your muscles to recuperate and avoid overtraining. Get enough sleep every night, as poor sleep might impair weight reduction and workout ability.

   On rest days, incorporate active recovery exercises like mild stretching, yoga, or low-intensity walks to help with blood flow and muscle healing. In conclusion, exercise and physical activity are essential components of a successful weight-loss regimen.

   On your weight reduction journey, combine cardiovascular exercise, strength training, flexibility and mobility exercises, and regular physical activity to increase calorie expenditure, build muscle, enhance cardiovascular health, and raise overall well-being.

Remember to personalize your workout regimen to your own fitness level, objectives, and tastes, and get advice from a healthcare practitioner or fitness expert if you have any concerns or medical issues. With persistence, perseverance, and a balanced approach to exercise, you may reach your weight reduction objectives while also reaping the numerous advantages of an active lifestyle. Importance of Exercise in Weight Loss

Importance of Exercise in Weight Loss

Starting Your Journey to Success Starting a weight reduction journey might be scary, but including exercise into your regimen is critical for long-term success.

Exercise aids in weight loss by burning calories, building muscle, improving metabolic health, and enhancing general well-being.

Let's look at the role of exercise in weight reduction and how it might help you start your road to a healthier, happier self.

1. Calorie expenditure: Exercise is one of the most efficient methods to generate a calorie deficit, which is required for weight loss. When you participate in physical exercise, your body burns calories for energy, which helps to maintain the overall energy balance required to reduce weight. By raising your activity level through exercise, you may raise your daily calorie expenditure and produce a larger calorie deficit, resulting in more weight reduction over time.

2. Muscle Building and Metabolic Boost: In addition to burning calories during exercise, including strength training in your regimen promotes lean muscle mass. Muscle tissue is metabolically active; therefore, it burns more calories at rest than fat tissue.

As you gain muscle mass through strength training activities, your resting metabolic rate rises, allowing you to burn more calories throughout the day, even when you are not exercising.

This metabolic boost can help you lose weight by raising your total calorie expenditure and encouraging fat loss.

3. Improved Metabolic Health: Regular exercise offers various metabolic advantages, including increased insulin sensitivity, blood sugar management, and lipid profile.

Exercise allows your body to use glucose more effectively, decreasing insulin resistance and lowering blood sugar levels.

It also accelerates the breakdown of triglycerides (a form of fat) and raises HDL cholesterol levels (the "good" cholesterol), which leads to better lipid profiles and a lower risk of cardiovascular disease. Exercise helps with weight loss and general well-being by boosting metabolism.

4. Appetite Regulation and Cravings: Exercise can help regulate appetite and reduce food cravings, making it simpler to stick to a calorie-controlled diet to lose weight. Physical exercise influences hunger and satiety hormones such as ghrelin and leptin. According to research, regular exercise may reduce levels of ghrelin (the hunger hormone) while increasing levels of leptin (the satiety hormone), resulting in fewer hunger pangs and better appetite control. Furthermore, exercise can help you avoid food cravings and provide a healthy coping mechanism for stress or emotional eating.

5. Mental and Emotional Wellbeing: In addition to its physical advantages, exercise has a significant impact on mental and emotional well-being, both of which are critical components of a successful weight reduction journey. Regular exercise releases endorphins, chemicals in the brain that increase happiness while reducing stress and anxiety. Exercise can also help with sleep quality, raise self-esteem and body image, and improve general happiness and quality of life. By including exercise in your weight reduction regimen, you can get mental and emotional advantages that promote long-term success and sustainability.

6. Long-term Weight Maintenance: Regular exercise is essential for long-term weight management after you've met your weight loss objectives. According to research, those who engage in regular physical exercise are more likely to sustain weight loss over time than those who are sedentary.

Exercise preserves lean muscle mass, prevents metabolic slowdown, and promotes a healthy body composition, making it simpler to maintain a low weight and avoid weight gain.

7. Enhancing Energy and Endurance: Regular exercise can boost your energy and stamina, making it simpler to complete everyday activities and physical responsibilities. As you increase your physical activity, your cardiovascular fitness and stamina improve, allowing you to do daily chores with less effort and tiredness. This improved energy and endurance can lead to a more active lifestyle, which can help you lose weight by pushing you to exercise more throughout the day.

8. Stress Reduction and Enhanced Coping Mechanisms: Exercise is an effective stress reliever and mood booster, providing a natural way to manage stress and improve emotional well-being.

Physical activity increases the synthesis of endorphins, chemicals in the brain that promote relaxation and enjoyment.

Regular exercise also reduces stress chemicals like cortisol, which can lead to overeating and weight gain.

Incorporating exercise into your weight reduction program will help you manage stress, enhance your mood, and create healthier coping skills that will benefit your overall health.

9. **Increasing Confidence and Self-Efficacy:** Regular exercise can help you gain confidence and self-efficacy, or belief in your capacity to achieve your goals. As you go through your fitness journey and reach milestones like improving strength, endurance, or flexibility, you will feel a sense of success and empowerment.

   This enhanced confidence and self-efficacy can extend beyond your exercise objectives and improve other aspects of your life, such as your ability to stick to a balanced diet, handle stress, and overcome obstacles on your weight loss path. 10.

10. Social Support and Accountability: Exercise allows you to interact with people and form social support networks, which can help with your weight reduction journey. Whether you attend a fitness class, participate in group exercises, or exercise with friends or family, having a supportive community may give you encouragement, accountability, and inspiration to stick to your exercise regimen.

Social support may also make exercise more fun and lasting, boosting the chances of long-term adherence and success in meeting your weight reduction objectives.

Exercise promotes weight loss in a variety of ways, including calorie expenditure, muscle strengthening, metabolic health, hunger management, mental and emotional well-being, energy levels, stress reduction, confidence, self-efficacy, and social support.

By combining a variety of physical activities into your routine, setting reasonable objectives, and making exercise a regular and pleasurable part of your daily routine, you may optimize the advantages of exercise and achieve long-term success in your weight reduction journey.

Remember that each step of physical activity puts you closer to your objectives, and with dedication and determination, you can alter your physique while also improving your entire health and well-being.

Choosing the Right Types of Exercise

Selecting the Right Types of Exercise When beginning a weight reduction regimen, selecting the appropriate sorts of exercise is critical for accomplishing your objectives successfully and safely. The appropriate combination of workouts can help you burn calories, gain muscle, enhance cardiovascular health, and improve your general well-being.

Here's how to pick the correct forms of exercise to help you lose weight:

1. Assess Your Fitness Level: Before deciding on a certain sort of exercise, you must first determine your present level of fitness. Consider your age, weight, health, and exercise history.

If you're new to exercising or have any underlying health concerns, speak with a healthcare expert or qualified fitness trainer to identify the best sorts of exercise for you.

2. Set realistic objectives: Consider your weight reduction objectives and how exercise might help you accomplish them. Whether you want to reduce weight, increase your fitness, or improve your general health, setting realistic and achievable objectives will help you choose workouts. Divide your objectives into smaller, more realistic milestones to keep yourself motivated and focused on success.

3. Consider Your Preferences and Interests: Select workouts you enjoy and look forward to completing. Finding activities that you love, such as dancing, cycling, swimming, hiking, or engaging in group fitness programs, will help you stay consistent and devoted to your workout regimen. Consider trying out several sorts of exercise to see what you love the best and what works into your schedule.

 4. Incorporate Variety: Incorporating a variety of exercises into your regimen helps minimize boredom, lower the chance of overuse injuries, and target different muscle groups for balanced fitness. Include a combination of cardiovascular exercise (e.g., walking, jogging, cycling, swimming), strength training (e.g., weightlifting, bodyweight exercises), flexibility and mobility exercises (e.g., yoga, Pilates, stretching), and functional movements (e.g., squats, lunges, core exercises).

5. Focus on full-body exercises: To increase calorie expenditure and muscle activation, focus on full-body exercises that target numerous muscle groups concurrently. Compound exercises, such as squats, deadlifts, push-ups, and rows, involve several joints and muscles, leading to more effective training and increased total calorie burn.

Incorporate functional motions that imitate real-life tasks to increase strength, stability, and mobility.

6. Gradually raise intensity: As you grow more acclimated to exercising, gradually raise the intensity of your exercises to continue pushing your body and making progress towards your goals. This might entail increasing the time or intensity of aerobic exercises, adding resistance or raising weights during strength training, or combining high-intensity interval training (HIIT) for a more intensive calorie burn.

7. Listen to Your Body: Pay attention to how your body responds to different forms of exercise and alter your regimen accordingly. If you encounter pain or discomfort during or after exercise, adjust or quit the activity, and check with a healthcare practitioner if necessary. Allow for adequate rest and recovery between workouts to prevent overtraining and promote muscle repair and growth.

8. Be consistent: Consistency is key to seeing results from your exercise routine. Aim to exercise regularly, ideally at least three to five days per week, to build momentum and progress towards your weight loss goals. Schedule workouts into your weekly routine and treat them as non-negotiable appointments with yourself. Remember that consistency over time is more important than occasional, intense workouts.

9. Track Your Progress: Keep track of your workouts, progress, and achievements to stay motivated and accountable. Whether you use a fitness tracker, smartphone app, journal, or simple spreadsheet, recording your workouts, duration, intensity, and any improvements can help you stay on track and celebrate your accomplishments along the way.

10. Stay Flexible and Adapt: Be flexible and willing to adapt your exercise routine as needed based on changes in your schedule, preferences, or goals. Life can be unpredictable, and it's important to find ways to stay active and maintain your exercise routine even during busy or challenging times. Be creative and find opportunities to incorporate physical activity into your daily life, whether it's taking the stairs instead of the elevator, going for a walk during your lunch break, or doing a quick home workout when time is limited.

By considering your fitness level, setting realistic goals, choosing activities you enjoy, incorporating variety, focusing on full-body workouts, gradually increasing intensity, listening to your body, being consistent, tracking your progress, and staying flexible and adaptable, you can choose the right types of exercise to kickstart your weight loss routine and achieve long-term success in your fitness journey.

Remember that exercise is not only about losing weight but also about improving your overall health, well-being, and quality of life. Enjoy the process, stay committed to your goals, and celebrate your progress along the way!

Creating a Sustainable Workout Routine

Building the Foundation for Long-Term Success in Your Weight Loss Journey When starting a weight loss routine, creating a sustainable workout routine is essential for achieving lasting results and maintaining a healthy lifestyle.

A sustainable workout routine is one that is enjoyable, flexible, and adaptable to your lifestyle, making it easier to stick with in the long run.

Here's how to create a sustainable workout routine to kickstart your weight loss journey:

1. Set realistic expectations: When designing your workout routine, set realistic expectations that align with your current fitness level, lifestyle, and weight loss goals. Avoid setting overly ambitious goals that may lead to burnout or disappointment. Instead, focus on gradual progress and celebrate small victories along the way.

2. Identify Your Motivation: Understand your reasons for wanting to lose weight and improve your fitness. Whether it's improving health markers, increasing energy levels, feeling more confident in your body, or simply enjoying the physical and mental benefits of exercise, identifying your motivation will help you stay committed to your workout routine during challenging times.

3. Choose Activities You Enjoy: Selecting activities that you genuinely enjoy is key to creating a sustainable workout routine. Whether it's walking, jogging, cycling, swimming, dancing, yoga, or strength training, choose activities that you look forward to and that fit your preferences and interests. Enjoying your workouts will make them feel less like a chore and more like a rewarding part of your day.

4. Prioritize Variety and Balance: Incorporate a variety of exercises and activities into your routine to prevent boredom, target different muscle groups, and improve overall fitness. Include cardiovascular exercise, strength training, flexibility and mobility exercises, and functional movements to create a well-rounded workout routine that promotes balanced fitness and overall health.

5. Start Slow and Gradually Increase Intensity: When beginning a new workout routine, start slow and gradually increase the intensity and duration of your workouts as your fitness level improves. Avoid the temptation to do too much too soon, as this can lead to fatigue, burnout, or injury. Listen to your body and progress at a pace that feels comfortable and sustainable for you.

6. Schedule Regular Workouts: Establish a consistent schedule for your workouts and treat them as non-negotiable appointments with yourself. Whether it's early morning, lunchtime, or evening, choose a time of day that works best for your schedule and stick to it. Consistency is key to developing a sustainable workout routine and seeing long-term results.

7. Be Flexible and Adapt: Life can be unpredictable, and it's important to be flexible and adaptable with your workout routine. If unexpected events or changes in your schedule disrupt your planned workouts, find alternative ways to stay active and move your body. Be creative and find opportunities to incorporate physical activity into your daily life, whether it's taking the stairs instead of the elevator, going for a walk during your lunch break, or doing a quick home workout when time is limited.

8. Listen to Your Body: Pay attention to how your body responds to exercise and adjust your routine accordingly. If you experience pain, fatigue, or discomfort during or after your workouts, modify or reduce the intensity or duration of your workouts as needed. Rest and recovery are essential components of a sustainable workout routine, so be sure to give your body adequate time to rest and repair between workouts.

9. Monitor Your Progress: Keep track of your workouts, progress, and achievements to stay motivated and accountable. Whether you use a fitness tracker, smartphone app, journal, or simple spreadsheet, recording your workouts, duration, intensity, and any improvements can help you stay on track and celebrate your accomplishments along the way.

10. Focus on Long-Term Health and Well-Being: Remember that weight loss is just one aspect of your overall health and well-being. Instead of focusing solely on the number on the scale, prioritize behaviors that promote long-term health and sustainable lifestyle changes.

Embrace the journey of self-improvement, celebrate your progress, and cultivate a positive mindset that supports your overall health and well-being.

By setting realistic expectations, identifying your motivation, choosing activities you enjoy, prioritizing variety and balance, starting slow and gradually increasing intensity, scheduling regular workouts, being flexible and adaptable, listening to your body, monitoring your progress, and focusing on long-term health and well-being, you can create a sustainable workout routine that supports your weight loss journey and leads to lasting success. Remember that consistency, patience, and self-care are key components of a sustainable lifestyle, and enjoy the journey as you work towards achieving your health and fitness goals.

"Building a sustainable workout routine is key to long-term success on your weight loss journey! 💪 Choose activities you enjoy, prioritize variety, and listen to your body. Consistency is key!#FitnessGoals"

Chapter 5: Lifestyle Modifications

Lifestyle changes are critical when starting a weight reduction journey because they address habits and behaviors that can have a substantial influence on your ability to attain and maintain a healthy weight.

Here's how lifestyle changes can help you start an effective weight-loss routine:

Dietary Changes: Eating a balanced and healthy diet is essential for losing weight. Include whole foods like fruits, vegetables, lean meats, whole grains, and healthy fats in your meals while limiting processed foods, sugary drinks, and high-calorie snacks. To avoid overeating, limit your meal sizes and practice mindful eating.

Meal Planning and Preparation: Preparing nutritious meals ahead of time will help you achieve your weight-reduction objectives. Set aside time each week to plan your meals, make a grocery list, and prep items in advance. Batch-preparing and portioning meals can help you save time and make healthy eating easier on hectic weekdays.

Mindful Eating: Consider your body's hunger and fullness signs, emotions, and surroundings when eating. Slow down and enjoy each bite, chew your meal fully, and minimize distractions like screens or multitasking. Mindful eating can help you build a healthy connection with food, avoid overeating, and feel more satisfied with meals.

Regular physical activity promotes weight loss and general health. Aim for at least 150 minutes of moderate-intensity aerobic activity or 75 minutes of vigorous-intensity aerobic exercise each week, as well as strength training activities targeting key muscle groups at least twice a week. Find activities you like and incorporate them into your normal schedule.

Stress Management: Long-term stress can lead to weight gain and hinder weight loss efforts. Incorporate stress-relieving hobbies like meditation, deep breathing exercises, yoga, or spending time outside into your daily routine. Prioritize self-care and schedule time for things that will help you relax and unwind, such as reading, bathing, or listening to music.

Adequate Sleep: Regular sleep is crucial for weight loss and general health. Aim for 7-9 hours of good sleep every night to help your body's natural activities, including metabolism, hormone management, and hunger control. Create a calm nighttime ritual, a pleasant sleeping environment, and prioritize consistency in your sleep pattern.

Hydration: Drinking enough water throughout the day promotes weight reduction and general wellness. Aim to drink 8–10 glasses of water each day, or more if you are physically active or in hot weather. Stay hydrated by carrying a reusable water bottle, setting reminders to drink water throughout the day, and including hydrating foods like fruits and vegetables in your meals.

Get assistance from friends, family, or peers to stay motivated on your weight reduction quest. Share your objectives with others, look for accountability partners, and join online or in-person support groups to meet like-minded people. A supportive network may offer encouragement, inspiration, and accountability as you try to achieve your weight reduction objectives.

Adopting behavior modification techniques can help overcome hurdles and create healthy behaviors for weight loss. Set precise, measurable, attainable, relevant, and time-bound (SMART) objectives, monitor your progress, identify triggers for harmful habits, and devise tactics to combat them. Practice self-compassion and resilience, and acknowledge your accomplishments along the way.

Prioritize long-term sustainability above short-term remedies or fad diets. Adopt a holistic approach to health and wellness that considers all parts of your life, such as diet, physical exercise, stress management, sleep, and social support.

Remember that little, persistent improvements over time can provide long-term effects and boost overall well-being. Lifestyle changes are essential for commencing an effective weight reduction regimen and achieving long-term outcomes.

You can create a healthy lifestyle that supports your weight loss goals and promotes overall well-being by incorporating healthy dietary habits, meal planning and preparation, mindful eating practices, regular physical activity, stress management techniques, adequate sleep, hydration, social support, behavior change strategies, and a focus on long-term sustainability.

Remember that every good adjustment you make helps you achieve your goals, and enjoy the path to a healthier, happier self.

Stress management techniques

Stress management is essential when starting a weight reduction program since it may have a big influence on your general well-being and weight control efforts. Implementing good stress management practices will help you deal with daily pressures, minimize emotional eating, and keep a positive attitude throughout your weight loss journey.

Here are some stress-management practices to consider incorporating into your routine.

1. Mindfulness Meditation: This practice effectively reduces tension and promotes relaxation. Spend a few minutes each day sitting quietly, focusing on your breath, and paying attention to the present moment. Notice any thoughts, feelings, or sensations without judgment and let them pass without attachment. Regular mindfulness meditation can help to relax the mind, reduce anxiety, and enhance general well-being.

2. Deep breathing activities: These activities promote relaxation and lessen tension. Practice diaphragmatic breathing by inhaling deeply with your nose, allowing your abdomen to expand, and gently expelling through your mouth, releasing tension with each breath. You can also practice progressive muscle relaxation, which involves tensing and relaxing different muscle groups in your body to relieve physical stress and promote relaxation.

3. Physical Activity: Regular physical activity helps reduce stress and enhance mood. Include enjoyable activities such as walking, running, cycling, dancing, or yoga in your everyday routine. Exercise helps to release endorphins, chemicals in the brain that increase happiness and reduce stress. Aim for at least 30 minutes of moderate-intensity exercise most days of the week to reap the stress-relieving effects.

4. Time Management: Organizing your everyday tasks helps lessen stress. Prioritize your duties and responsibilities, establish realistic goals, and divide bigger tasks into smaller, more manageable steps. Schedule your time using tools like calendars, planners, or smartphone applications, and make sure you leave enough time for work, exercise, leisure, and socializing. Setting limits and learning to say no to non-essential obligations can also help you minimize stress and avoid overwhelm.

5. Healthy lifestyle behaviors: Practicing healthy behaviors can improve stress management and well-being. Ensure that you receive enough sleep each night, aiming for 7-9 hours of quality sleep, since a lack of sleep can worsen stress. To promote good physical and mental health, eat a well-balanced diet rich in fruits and vegetables, whole grains, lean proteins, and healthy fats. Limit your use of coffee, alcohol, and sugary meals, since these can all lead to increased tension and anxiety.

6. Social Support: Connecting with supportive friends, family, or peers can offer emotional support and relieve stress. Share your thoughts and experiences with trusted people, and seek their advice or perspectives as required. Participate in social activities, support groups, or community events to build a sense of belonging and connection. Spending time with loved ones and participating in fun social activities might help reduce stress and enhance mood.

7. Incorporate relaxation techniques into your regular practice to reduce stress. Practice things such as reading, listening to music, having a warm bath, going for a walk in nature, or indulging in hobbies that you enjoy. Find activities that help you rest and rejuvenate, and schedule them on a regular basis to improve your general well-being.

8. Positive Self-Talk: Develop a positive mentality and use positive self-talk to manage stress and resilience. Challenge negative thoughts and replace them with more positive, inspiring words. Concentrate on your talents, accomplishments, and development, and recognize your efforts and successes along the way.

Adopting a growth mindset and seeing problems as chances for development might help you deal with stress more successfully. Incorporating stress management tactics into your weight reduction regimen is critical for maintaining general well-being and attaining lasting results. Mindfulness meditation, deep breathing exercises, physical activity, time management, healthy lifestyle habits, social support, relaxation techniques, and positive self-talk can all help you manage stress, reduce emotional eating, and maintain a positive mindset during your weight loss journey.

Remember to emphasize self-care, listen to your body's demands, and be kind to yourself as you go through the ups and downs of your weight-loss journey.

Improving sleep quality

Improving sleep quality is a crucial aspect of starting a successful weight loss routine, as adequate sleep plays a significant role in regulating hormones, metabolism, and appetite. Poor sleep quality can disrupt these processes, leading to increased cravings for high-calorie foods, decreased energy levels, and hindered weight-loss efforts. Here are some strategies to help you improve sleep quality and support your weight loss journey:

1. Establish a consistent sleep schedule. Try to go to bed and wake up at the same time every day, even on weekends. Consistency in your sleep schedule helps regulate your body's internal clock, making it easier to fall asleep and wake up naturally. Aim for 7-9 hours of quality sleep each night to support your overall health and well-being.

2. Create a Relaxing Bedtime Routine: Develop a relaxing bedtime routine to signal to your body that it's time to wind down and prepare for sleep. Activities such as reading, taking a warm bath, practicing gentle yoga or meditation, or listening to soothing music can help relax your mind and body and promote better sleep quality. Avoid stimulating activities or screens (e.g., smartphones, computers, TVs) close to bedtime, as they can interfere with your ability to fall asleep.

3. Create a Comfortable Sleep Environment: Create a comfortable and conducive sleep environment to promote better sleep quality. Make sure your bedroom is cool, dark, and quiet, and invest in a comfortable mattress and pillows that support your body. Use blackout curtains or an eye mask to block out light, and consider using white noise machines or earplugs to mask any disruptive noises.

4. Limit Stimulants and Electronics Before Bed: Avoid consuming stimulants such as caffeine and nicotine in the hours leading up to bedtime, as they can interfere with your ability to fall asleep. Avoid exposing yourself to the blue light emitted from electronic devices with screens, such as smartphones, tablets, and computers, as it can suppress the production of melatonin, a hormone that regulates sleep-wake cycles.

5. Practice stress reduction techniques: Stress and anxiety can interfere with sleep quality, so it's essential to practice stress reduction techniques to promote relaxation and better sleep. Engage in activities that help you unwind and de-stress, such as deep breathing exercises, progressive muscle relaxation, guided imagery, or journaling. Find what works best for you and incorporate these techniques into your daily routine to improve sleep quality and overall well-being. 6. Exercise Regularly, But Not Too Close to Bedtime: Regular physical activity can improve sleep quality by promoting relaxation and reducing stress and anxiety. However, it's essential to avoid vigorous exercise too close to bedtime, as it can have a stimulating effect and make it harder to fall asleep. Aim to finish your workout at least a few hours before bedtime to allow your body time to wind down and prepare for sleep.

7. Watch Your Diet and Hydration: Be mindful of your diet and hydration habits, as they can affect your sleep quality. Avoid heavy meals, spicy foods, and excessive fluid intake close to bedtime, as they can cause discomfort and disrupt sleep. Instead, opt for light, balanced meals and limit caffeine and alcohol consumption, especially in the evening, as they can interfere with sleep patterns.

8. Seek Professional Help if Needed: If you continue to struggle with sleep despite implementing these strategies, consider seeking professional help from a healthcare provider or sleep specialist. They can help identify any underlying sleep disorders or issues contributing to poor sleep quality and provide personalized recommendations or treatment options to improve your sleep. Improving sleep quality is a crucial component of starting a successful weight-loss routine.

By prioritizing sleep hygiene, establishing a consistent sleep schedule, creating a relaxing bedtime routine, optimizing your sleep environment, limiting stimulants and electronics before bed, practicing stress reduction techniques, exercising regularly, watching your diet and hydration, and seeking professional help if needed, you can support your overall health and well-being and enhance your weight loss efforts.

Remember that quality sleep is essential for physical, mental, and emotional health, and prioritizing sleep can positively impact every aspect of your life.

Strategies for Overcoming Plateaus

When starting a weight loss routine, it's common to encounter plateaus—periods where your weight loss stalls despite your continued efforts. Plateaus can be frustrating and demotivating, but they are a natural part of the weight-loss process. Fortunately, there are several strategies you can employ to overcome plateaus and continue making progress towards your goals:

1. **Reassess Your Caloric Intake:** As you lose weight, your body's caloric needs may change, leading to a decrease in metabolic rate. To overcome a plateau, reassess your caloric intake and adjust as necessary.

   Consider recalculating your daily calorie needs based on your current weight, activity level, and goals. Use a food diary or tracking app to monitor your intake and ensure you're in a calorie deficit while still meeting your nutritional needs.

2. **Increase Physical Activity:** If you've reached a plateau, increasing your physical activity can help kick-start your weight loss again. Incorporate more exercise into your routine by adding extra workouts, increasing the intensity or duration of your workouts, or trying new activities that challenge your body in different ways. Including both cardiovascular exercise and strength training can help maximize calorie burn and build lean muscle mass, which can boost your metabolism.

3. **Mix Up Your Workouts:** Variety is key to overcoming plateaus in your weight loss routine. If

you've been doing the same workouts for an extended period, your body may have adapted to the routine, leading to diminished results. Mix up your workouts by trying new exercises, changing the order or intensity of your workouts, or incorporating different types of exercise modalities, such as interval training, circuit training, or high-intensity interval training (HIIT). Adding variety can shock your body and prevent it from reaching a plateau.

4. **Focus on Strength Training:** Strength training is an effective way to overcome plateaus and break through weight loss stalls. Building lean muscle mass through strength training can increase your metabolic rate, allowing you to burn more calories at rest. Aim to incorporate strength training exercises that target all major muscle groups at least two to three times per week. Progressive overload, or gradually increasing the weight or resistance you lift over time, can help stimulate muscle growth and further boost your metabolism.

5. **Prioritize Recovery and Sleep:** Adequate rest and recovery are essential for overcoming plateaus and

supporting weight loss. Make sure you're getting enough quality sleep each night, as sleep deprivation can disrupt hormone levels and metabolism, making weight loss more challenging. Incorporate rest days into your workout routine to allow your body to recover and repair muscle tissue. Manage stress through relaxation techniques such as meditation, deep breathing exercises, or gentle yoga to support overall well-being and promote recovery.

6. **Monitor non-scale victories:** Progress may not always be reflected on the scale, but that doesn't mean you're not making strides in other areas. Monitor non-scale victories such as improvements in strength, endurance, energy levels, mood, and clothing fit to stay motivated and focused on your overall progress. Celebrate these achievements as signs of success on your weight loss journey, even if the scale isn't moving as quickly as you'd like.

7. **Stay consistent and patient:** Consistency and patience are key when overcoming plateaus in your weight loss routine. Remember that weight loss is not always linear, and progress may come in fits

and starts. Stay committed to your healthy habits, trust the process, and be patient with yourself as you work towards your goals. Focus on making sustainable lifestyle changes that support long-term success rather than quick fixes or drastic measures. By reassessing your caloric intake, increasing physical activity, mixing up your workouts, focusing on strength training, prioritizing recovery and sleep, monitoring non-scale victories, staying consistent, and being patient, you can overcome plateaus in your weight loss routine and continue making progress towards your goals. Remember that plateaus are a normal part of the journey, and with perseverance and determination, you can break through barriers and achieve lasting success.

Chapter 6: Long-term Maintenance and Sustainability.

Long-term Maintenance and Sustainability: The Key to Permanent Weight Loss Success

Starting a weight reduction regimen is frequently the first step toward accomplishing your health and fitness objectives, but the true issue is keeping up your progress over time. Long-term maintenance and sustainability are critical components of any weight reduction journey, ensuring that you not only achieve your goal weight but also maintain it for the rest of your life. Here are some key methods to help you attain long-term success and sustainability in your weight reduction regimen:

1. Build practical and sustainable behaviors: When starting a weight reduction journey, it's crucial to create behaviors that are both practical and long-lasting. Avoid severe or restrictive diets that are difficult to stick to over time, instead focusing on making incremental, long-term improvements to your eating habits and lifestyle. Choose nutrient-dense, whole foods that you love and include them in your regular meals in a way that suits your needs and lifestyle.

2. Maintaining a healthy weight requires balance and moderation in your eating habits and lifestyle. Allow yourself to eat your favorite foods in moderation rather than categorizing them as "off-limits" or "forbidden." Practice mindful eating by paying attention to your body's hunger and fullness cues, enabling yourself to indulge periodically without guilt. By establishing balance and moderation, you may eat a broad range of meals while still losing weight.

3. Prioritize Behavior Change: Rather than focusing simply on the scale, establish healthy habits that promote long-term well-being. Determine which actions and habits have contributed to your weight reduction achievement and attempt to reinforce them over time. Whether it's portion control, meal planning, physical activity, or stress management, cultivate beneficial behaviors that benefit your overall health and weight management.

4. Maintain Healthy Habits: Consistency is essential for long-term weight management and sustainability. Make healthy food and frequent physical exercise a part of your daily routine, even after you've met your weight reduction targets. Set reasonable objectives for yourself and stick to them over time, especially when confronted with obstacles or failures. Consistency in your behaviors will allow you to retain your success and avoid weight gain in the long run.

5. Prioritize Self-Care and Stress Management: Ensuring your physical, mental, and emotional well-being is crucial for long-term weight reduction success. Prioritize self-care activities that help you manage stress, relax, and recharge, such as mindfulness meditation, participating in hobbies you like, spending time with loved ones, or going outside in nature. Managing stress efficiently can help you avoid emotional eating and improve your overall health and well-being.

6. Maintain Flexibility and Adaptability: To successfully lose weight, it's important to be adaptive to life's unforeseen obstacles. Be prepared to modify your food habits and exercise regimen to fit changes in your schedule, preferences, or situation. Adopt a flexible mentality and be open to trying new techniques or approaches in order to continue your development and achieve long-term success.

7. Seek Support and Accountability: Having a support network of friends, family, or peers may offer encouragement, inspiration, and accountability during your weight reduction journey. Share your objectives with others and ask them to help you remain on track. Consider joining a weight reduction support group, hiring a personal trainer, or teaming up with an exercise companion to stay motivated and accountable.

8. Recognize and appreciate non-scale accomplishments alongside weight loss milestones. Celebrate the good changes you've seen as a consequence of your weight loss journey, whether they're in your energy levels, happiness, fitness, or general health. Focusing on non-scale wins will keep you motivated and encouraged to make long-term, healthy decisions.

Incorporating these tactics into your daily routine will not only help you lose weight but will also encourage long-term maintenance and sustainability. Remember that keeping a healthy weight is more than just achieving a specific number on the scale; it is also about living a balanced and meaningful lifestyle that promotes your entire well-being.

1. Be Mindful of Your Eating Habits: Mindful eating entails paying attention to your food selections, eating carefully, and appreciating every mouthful. Being conscious of your eating patterns allows you to better tune into your body's hunger and fullness cues, which prevents overeating and promotes a balanced connection with food.

2. Remain Active: Regular physical exercise is critical for sustaining weight reduction and general health. Find activities you like and incorporate them into your normal schedule. Staying active, whether through walking, bicycling, swimming, or group exercise courses, can help you burn calories, gain strength, and improve your mood.

3. Monitor Your Progress: Keep track of your progress by periodically checking your weight, measurements, and other health and fitness markers. This will keep you accountable and motivated, allowing you to make changes to your routine as necessary.

4. Practice self-compassion: Be gentle with yourself during your weight reduction journey. Remember that failures and obstacles are a normal part of the process, and you should treat yourself with kindness and understanding. Instead of concentrating on mistakes or failures, consider how you may learn from them.

5. Stay Connected: Surround yourself with friends, family, and peers who understand and support your weight reduction objectives. Share your accomplishments and struggles with them, and rely on them for assistance when necessary. Having a solid support system may help you stay motivated and committed.

6. Be Patient and Persistent: Remember that lasting weight reduction requires time, patience, and perseverance. It is natural to have variations in weight and progress along the road, but it is critical to keep focused on your long-term objectives. Trust the process, stick to your healthy habits, and enjoy minor victories along the way.

7. Celebrate Your Achievements: As you progress through your weight reduction journey, take time to recognize your accomplishments and milestones. Whether it's attaining a specific weight or clothing size, finishing a difficult workout, or setting a personal best, enjoy your accomplishments and recognize the hard work and devotion required to get there.

8. Seek Professional Guidance if Needed: If you're having trouble maintaining your weight reduction or encountering difficulties along the road, don't be afraid to seek professional help from a healthcare physician, registered nutritionist, or certified personal trainer. They can provide specialized guidance, assistance, and resources to help you overcome hurdles and stay on track with your objectives.

Long-term maintenance and sustainability are critical components of any effective weight loss program. You can achieve long-term success in your weight loss journey by establishing realistic and sustainable habits, finding balance and moderation, focusing on behavior change, sticking to healthy habits, prioritizing self-care and stress management, remaining flexible and adaptable, seeking support and accountability, and celebrating non-scale victories. Remember that losing weight is a journey, not a destination, and put your entire health and well-being first.

Setbacks

Embarking on a weight loss routine is an empowering decision towards improving your health and well-being. However, along the journey, you may encounter setbacks and challenges that can test your resolve and commitment.

Handling these setbacks and challenges effectively is crucial for staying motivated and continuing towards your weight loss goals.

First and foremost, it's essential to acknowledge that setbacks and challenges are a normal part of any transformative journey, including weight loss.

Rather than viewing them as failures, see them as opportunities for growth and learning. Remember that progress is not always linear, and it's okay to experience bumps along the way.

One of the most important strategies for handling setbacks and challenges is to maintain a positive mindset. Instead of dwelling on setbacks or feeling discouraged, focus on what you can learn from the experience and how you can use it to propel yourself forward. Cultivate self-compassion and kindness toward yourself, recognizing that setbacks are a natural part of the process.

It's also essential to stay flexible and adaptable in your approach to weight loss. If a particular strategy or routine isn't working for you, don't be afraid to reassess and make adjustments as needed. Be open to trying new approaches, seeking advice from professionals, or seeking support from friends and family.

Another key aspect of handling setbacks and challenges is to practice resilience. Resilience involves bouncing back from setbacks and adversity and staying committed to your goals despite obstacles.

Cultivate resilience by focusing on your strengths, maintaining a sense of purpose, and reminding yourself of your reasons for wanting to lose weight. When faced with challenges, it's crucial to have a plan in place for how you will overcome them. Identify potential obstacles that may arise on your weight loss journey, such as cravings, busy schedules, or social events, and develop strategies for addressing them. This may include finding healthier alternatives to your favorite foods, scheduling workouts in advance, or practicing stress management techniques. Seeking support from others can also be instrumental in overcoming setbacks and challenges.

Overcoming Setbacks

Surround yourself with positive influences who understand and support your weight-loss goals. Share your struggles and victories with friends, family members, or support groups that can offer encouragement, advice, and accountability. Remember to celebrate your successes, no matter how small. Recognize and acknowledge your progress along the way, whether it's reaching a milestone, sticking to your healthy habits, or overcoming a challenge. Celebrating your achievements can boost your confidence and motivations, helping you stay focused on your long-term goals.

Handling setbacks and challenges is an integral part of starting a weight-loss routine. By maintaining a positive mindset, staying flexible and adaptable, practicing resilience, having a plan in place, seeking support from others, and celebrating your successes, you can overcome obstacles and continue towards your weight loss goals with confidence and determination. Remember that setbacks are temporary, but your commitment to your health and well-being is enduring.

Celebrating Successes

Celebrating successes and staying motivated are crucial components of starting a weight-loss routine and achieving long-term success.

As you embark on your journey to better health and well-being, it's essential to recognize and acknowledge your accomplishments, no matter how small, and to stay inspired and motivated along the way.

It's important to celebrate your successes, no matter how big or small. Whether you've reached a milestone in your weight-loss journey, made healthier food choices, or completed a challenging workout, take the time to acknowledge and celebrate your achievements.

Celebrating your successes not only boosts your confidence and self-esteem but also reinforces positive behaviors and motivates you to continue making progress.

In addition to celebrating your successes, it's essential to stay motivated and inspired throughout your weight-loss journey. One way to stay motivated is to set specific, measurable, achievable, relevant, and time-bound (SMART) goals for you. These goals give you a clear direction and something to strive for, helping you stay focused and motivated. Another effective strategy for staying motivated is to find sources of inspiration and support.

Surround yourself with positive influences that encourage and support your weight loss goals, whether it's friends, family members, or online communities. Share your successes and challenges with others who understand and can offer encouragement, advice, and accountability.

Additionally, find ways to reward yourself for your hard work and dedication. Treat yourself to non-food rewards, such as a relaxing spa day, a new workout outfit, or a fun activity you enjoy.

These rewards not only serve as incentives to stay motivated but also provide a sense of accomplishment and satisfaction. It's also essential to stay focused on the reasons why you started your weight-loss journey in the first place.

Whether it's improving your health, boosting your confidence, or setting a positive example for your loved ones, keeping your goals and motivations in mind can help you stay committed and driven, even when faced with challenges.

Track your progress along the way to stay motivated and inspired. Keep a journal or use a fitness tracking app to record your workouts, meals, and progress towards your goals. Seeing how far you've come can be incredibly motivating and remind you of the progress you've made, even on days when you feel discouraged.

Remember to be kind to yourself and practice self-compassion throughout your weight-loss journey. Setbacks and challenges are a natural part of the process, and it's essential to treat yourself with kindness and understanding during these times. Instead of dwelling on setbacks, focus on what you can learn from them and use them as opportunities for growth and improvement.

Celebrating successes and staying motivated are essential aspects of starting a weight-loss routine and achieving long-term success. By acknowledging and celebrating your accomplishments, setting SMART goals, finding sources of inspiration and support, rewarding yourself for your hard work, staying focused on your motivations, tracking your progress, and practicing self-compassion, you can stay motivated and inspired on your journey towards better health and well-being.

Remember that every step forward, no matter how small, is a step in the right direction, and celebrate your progress along the way.